Chapter 1: Introduction to the 30-Day Weight Management Challenge

Understanding the Importance of Weight Management

Welcome to the subchapter on "Understanding the Importance of Weight Management" in our book, "The 30-Day Weight Management Challenge: A Guide for Men and Women Aged 20-50." In this section, we will explore why weight management is crucial for your overall health and well-being, and how it can positively impact your life.

Maintaining a healthy weight is not just about looking good, it's about feeling good too. Excess weight can put a strain on your heart, joints, and overall health, leading to a variety of health issues such as heart disease, diabetes, and high blood pressure. By managing your weight effectively, you can reduce your risk of these conditions and increase your overall quality of life.

Weight management is also important for boosting your energy levels and improving your mood. When you carry excess weight, you may feel sluggish and tired, making it difficult to stay active and engaged in your daily activities. By maintaining a healthy weight, you can increase your energy levels and feel more positive and motivated in your daily life.

In addition to the physical benefits of weight management, there are also mental and emotional benefits to consider. Research has shown that maintaining a healthy weight can improve your self-esteem and confidence, leading to a more positive self-image and outlook on life. By taking control of your weight and making healthy choices, you can feel more empowered and in control of your overall well-being.

Overall, understanding the importance of weight management is crucial for your long-term health and happiness. By making small changes to your lifestyle and implementing healthy habits, you can achieve and maintain a healthy weight that will benefit you in countless ways. Remember, it's never too late to start prioritizing your health and well-being – you have the power to take control of your weight and live a happier, healthier life.

Setting Realistic Goals for the Challenge

Setting realistic goals for the challenge is crucial to your success in the 30-Day Weight Management Challenge. As men and women aged 20 to 50, it's important to understand that sustainable weight loss takes time and patience. By setting realistic goals, you can avoid feeling overwhelmed and increase your chances of achieving long-term success.

When setting your goals, it's important to be specific and measurable. Instead of saying, "I want to lose weight," try setting a specific goal like, "I want to lose 5 pounds in the next 30 days." This gives you a clear target to aim for and allows you to track your progress along the way. By breaking your larger goal into smaller, more manageable steps, you can stay motivated and focused throughout the challenge.

It's also important to set goals that are attainable and realistic. While it's great to have ambitious goals, setting goals that are too far out of reach can lead to frustration and disappointment. Instead, focus on setting goals that are challenging but achievable. For example, if you currently don't exercise at all, setting a goal to work out five days a week may be too ambitious. Start with smaller goals, such as exercising for 30 minutes three times a week, and gradually increase from there.

In addition to setting specific, measurable, attainable, and realistic goals, it's important to set a timeline for achieving them. By giving yourself a deadline, you create a sense of urgency and accountability that can help keep you on track. However, it's important to be flexible with your timeline and adjust as needed. If you don't reach your goal by the end of the 30 days, don't get discouraged. Use it as an opportunity to reassess your strategy and set new goals for the next month.

Remember, the 30-Day Weight Management Challenge is not just about reaching a number on the scale. It's about creating healthy habits that will last a lifetime. By setting realistic goals and staying focused on your progress, you can make lasting changes to your lifestyle and achieve your weight management goals. Stay positive, stay motivated, and most importantly, stay committed to the challenge. You've got this!

How This Book Will Help You Achieve Your Goals

Are you tired of struggling with your weight and feeling like you'll never reach your goals? If so, this book is here to offer you the guidance and support you need to finally take control of your health and achieve the results you've been dreaming of. The 30-Day Weight Management Challenge is specifically designed for men and women aged 20-50 who are ready to commit to making positive changes in their lives.

This book will help you achieve your goals by providing you with a comprehensive plan that covers everything from nutrition and exercise to mindset and motivation. You'll learn how to set realistic and achievable goals, create a sustainable meal plan, and incorporate regular physical activity into your routine. By following the step-by-step guidance outlined in this book, you'll be well on your way to reaching your weight management goals in just 30 days.

One of the key benefits of this book is that it takes a holistic approach to weight management, focusing not just on the physical aspects of health, but also on the mental and emotional components. You'll learn how to overcome common obstacles such as stress eating, emotional eating, and negative self-talk, so you can develop a healthier relationship with food and your body. By addressing these underlying issues, you'll be better equipped to stay on track and maintain your progress long-term.

In addition to practical tips and strategies, this book also offers plenty of encouragement and motivation to keep you inspired throughout the 30-day challenge. You'll find inspiring success stories from real men and women who have transformed their bodies and lives through similar programs, as well as uplifting quotes and affirmations to help you stay positive and focused. With the support of this book and the community of like-minded individuals embarking on the challenge alongside you, you'll never feel alone in your journey towards better health and wellness.

So if you're ready to finally take charge of your weight and achieve the results you've always wanted, this book is the perfect tool to help you get there. By committing to the 30-Day Weight Management Challenge and following the guidance provided within these pages, you'll not only reach your goals, but you'll also develop the skills and habits necessary to maintain a healthy lifestyle for years to come. Don't wait any longer – start your journey today and see the amazing transformation that awaits you!

Chapter 2: Preparing for the Challenge

Evaluating Your Current Eating Habits

In order to successfully manage your weight, it is crucial to evaluate your current eating habits. This subchapter will guide you through the process of assessing your diet and making necessary changes to support your weight management goals. By taking a closer look at what you eat on a daily basis, you will be able to identify areas for improvement and implement healthier choices that will benefit your overall well-being.

First and foremost, it is important to track your food intake for a few days to get a clear picture of your eating habits. This can be done by keeping a food journal or using a mobile app to record everything you consume throughout the day. By documenting your meals and snacks, you will be able to see patterns in your eating behaviors and identify areas where you may be overindulging or lacking in essential nutrients. This self-awareness is the first step towards making positive changes to your diet.

Next, take a closer look at the types of foods you are consuming on a regular basis. Are you eating a variety of fruits, vegetables, whole grains, lean proteins, and healthy fats? Or are you relying on processed foods, sugary snacks, and fast food for the majority of your meals? Evaluating the quality of your diet will help you determine if you are getting the nutrients your body needs to function optimally. Making small changes, such as adding more vegetables to your plate or swapping out sugary drinks for water, can have a big impact on your overall health and weight management goals.

In addition to assessing the types of foods you are eating, it is also important to consider your portion sizes and eating habits. Are you eating large portions at every meal, even when you are not hungry? Do you find yourself mindlessly snacking throughout the day, even when you are not hungry? By paying attention to your portion sizes and eating cues, you can avoid overeating and make more mindful choices when it comes to food. Eating slowly, savoring each bite, and listening to your body's hunger and fullness cues can help you develop a healthier relationship with food and support your weight management efforts.

Finally, it is essential to evaluate your emotional relationship with food. Do you turn to food for comfort, stress relief, or boredom? Are you prone to emotional eating or using food as a coping mechanism for difficult emotions? By recognizing your emotional triggers and finding alternative ways to cope with stress or negative emotions, you can break free from unhealthy eating patterns and develop a more balanced approach to food. Remember, it is okay to enjoy your favorite foods in moderation, but it is important to be mindful of your reasons for eating and make choices that support your overall health and well-being. By evaluating your current eating habits and making small, sustainable changes, you can set yourself up for success on your weight management journey.

Clearing Out Temptations in Your Kitchen

Clearing out temptations in your kitchen is an essential step in achieving your weight management goals. It's easy to give in to cravings when unhealthy snacks and treats are readily available. By removing these temptations from your kitchen, you can create a more supportive environment for making healthier choices.

Start by taking a good look at what's currently in your pantry and fridge. Are there any foods that are high in sugar, fat, or calories that you tend to reach for when you're feeling hungry or stressed? Consider getting rid of these items or replacing them with healthier alternatives. By clearing out these temptations, you'll be less likely to indulge in unhealthy eating habits.

One strategy for clearing out temptations in your kitchen is to make a list of the foods you want to avoid and then systematically remove them from your home. This might involve throwing away junk food, donating unopened items to a food pantry, or giving them to a friend or family member. Be ruthless in your approach and remember that you're doing this for your own well-being.

As you clear out temptations in your kitchen, consider replacing them with nutritious options that will support your weight management goals. Stock up on fruits, vegetables, whole grains, lean proteins, and other healthy snacks that you enjoy. Having these items on hand will make it easier to resist the temptation of reaching for unhealthy foods when hunger strikes.

Remember, clearing out temptations in your kitchen is just one step in your weight management journey. Stay committed to making healthy choices, staying active, and seeking support from friends, family, or a professional if needed. By creating a supportive environment in your home, you'll be setting yourself up for success in reaching your weight management goals.

Creating a Meal Plan for the 30 Days

Congratulations on taking the first step towards achieving your weight management goals! Creating a meal plan for the next 30 days is a crucial component of your journey towards a healthier lifestyle. By planning out your meals in advance, you can ensure that you are making nutritious choices that will support your weight management efforts.

When creating a meal plan for the next 30 days, it's important to consider your individual dietary needs and preferences. Start by taking an inventory of the foods you enjoy and the ones that will help you reach your weight management goals. Incorporate a variety of fruits, vegetables, lean proteins, whole grains, and healthy fats into your meal plan to ensure you are getting all the essential nutrients your body needs.

In addition to choosing nutrient-dense foods, be mindful of portion sizes when creating your meal plan. It's easy to overeat when faced with large portions, so aim to include balanced meals that are satisfying but not excessive. Consider using measuring cups or a food scale to help you portion out your meals and snacks to avoid overeating.

To make meal planning easier, consider batch cooking and meal prepping for the week ahead. By preparing meals in advance, you can save time and ensure that you always have healthy options available when hunger strikes. Choose recipes that are easy to make in bulk and can be stored in the fridge or freezer for later use.

Lastly, don't forget to listen to your body and make adjustments to your meal plan as needed. If you find that you are constantly hungry or lacking energy, it may be a sign that you need to adjust your portion sizes or add more nutrient-dense foods to your plan. Remember, this is a journey towards better health, and it's important to be flexible and make changes as you learn what works best for your body.

Chapter 3: Getting Started with Exercise

Finding an Exercise Routine That Works for You

Finding an exercise routine that works for you is crucial when it comes to achieving your weight management goals. It's important to remember that what works for one person may not work for another, so it's essential to find an exercise routine that fits your lifestyle and preferences. Whether you enjoy running, cycling, yoga, or weightlifting, there are countless options to choose from. The key is to find something you enjoy, so you'll be more likely to stick with it in the long run.

When selecting an exercise routine, consider your schedule and commitments. If you have a busy lifestyle, you may need to find a routine that can be done in a short amount of time, such as high-intensity interval training (HIIT) workouts. On the other hand, if you have more flexibility in your schedule, you may opt for longer, more leisurely workouts. The important thing is to find a routine that you can realistically commit to on a regular basis.

It's also important to consider your fitness level when choosing an exercise routine. If you're just starting out, you may want to begin with low-impact exercises and gradually increase the intensity as your fitness improves. On the other hand, if you're already in good shape, you may want to challenge yourself with more intense workouts. Remember, it's okay to start slow and build up your fitness level over time.

In addition to finding an exercise routine that you enjoy and can commit to, it's important to listen to your body and make adjustments as needed. If you're feeling fatigued or experiencing pain, it's important to take a break and rest. Pushing yourself too hard can lead to injury and setbacks in your weight management journey. Remember, progress takes time, so be patient with yourself and focus on making small, sustainable changes.

In conclusion, finding an exercise routine that works for you is essential for achieving your weight management goals. By considering your preferences, schedule, fitness level, and listening to your body, you can create a routine that will help you reach your desired outcomes. Remember, consistency is key, so find something you enjoy and can stick with in the long term. With dedication and perseverance, you can achieve success in your weight management journey.

Incorporating Strength Training and Cardio

Incorporating strength training and cardio into your weight management routine is essential for achieving long-lasting results. Strength training helps build muscle mass, which in turn increases your metabolism and helps you burn more calories throughout the day. Cardio, on the other hand, helps improve your cardiovascular health and burns calories quickly, leading to weight loss.

When combining strength training and cardio, it's important to find a balance that works for you. Aim to incorporate both types of exercise into your routine at least three to four times a week. This will help you build muscle, burn fat, and improve your overall fitness level. Remember, consistency is key when it comes to seeing results, so make sure to stick to your workout schedule.

One way to incorporate strength training and cardio into your routine is by alternating days. For example, you could do strength training exercises on Monday, Wednesday, and Friday, and cardio on Tuesday and Thursday. This will give your muscles time to recover between workouts while still allowing you to stay active and burn calories.

Another option is to combine strength training and cardio into one workout session. This can be done by incorporating circuit training, which involves performing a series of strength exercises followed by cardio intervals. This type of workout is efficient and effective, as it helps you build strength while also getting your heart rate up.

Overall, incorporating strength training and cardio into your weight management routine is crucial for achieving your fitness goals. By finding a balance that works for you and staying consistent with your workouts, you will be on your way to a healthier, stronger, and more fit version of yourself. Remember, progress takes time, so be patient with yourself and trust the process.

Tracking Your Progress and Making Adjustments

Congratulations on taking the first step towards a healthier lifestyle by embarking on the 30-Day Weight Management Challenge! As you continue on this journey, it is important to track your progress and make adjustments along the way to ensure that you are on the right path towards reaching your goals.

One of the most effective ways to track your progress is by keeping a food and exercise journal. By writing down everything you eat and tracking your physical activity, you will be able to see patterns and identify areas where you can make improvements. This simple yet powerful tool will help you stay accountable and make informed decisions about your health and wellness.

In addition to keeping a journal, it is important to regularly weigh yourself and take measurements of your body. While the number on the scale is not the only indicator of progress, it can be a helpful tool to track changes in your weight over time. Taking measurements of your waist, hips, and other key areas will also give you a more comprehensive view of your progress.

As you track your progress, it is important to be honest with yourself and make adjustments as needed. If you find that you are not seeing the results you desire, take a closer look at your diet and exercise routine. Are there areas where you can make healthier choices or increase your physical activity? By making small changes and being consistent, you will be able to see improvements in your overall health and well-being.

Remember, progress is not always linear, and there will be ups and downs along the way. Stay positive, stay focused, and keep pushing forward towards your goals. By tracking your progress and making adjustments as needed, you will be well on your way to achieving lasting weight management success.

Chapter 4: Exploring Weight Management Products

Understanding the Different Types of Weight Management Products

In order to successfully navigate the world of weight management products, it is essential to understand the different types available on the market. By familiarizing yourself with the various options, you can make informed decisions about which products may best suit your individual needs and goals. From supplements to meal replacement shakes, there is a wide range of products designed to assist you on your weight management journey.

One common type of weight management product is supplements. These can come in the form of vitamins, minerals, herbs, or other substances that are intended to support weight loss efforts. It is important to research the ingredients in any supplement you are considering, as some may have side effects or interactions with other medications. Additionally, supplements should be used in conjunction with a healthy diet and exercise routine for best results.

Meal replacement shakes are another popular option for those looking to manage their weight. These shakes typically contain a balance of protein, carbohydrates, and fats, as well as essential vitamins and minerals. They can be a convenient option for busy individuals who may not have time to prepare a nutritious meal. However, it is important to choose a meal replacement shake that is low in sugar and high in protein to keep you feeling full and satisfied.

Another type of weight management product is appetite suppressants. These products work by reducing feelings of hunger, making it easier to stick to a calorie-controlled diet. While appetite suppressants can be helpful for some individuals, it is important to use them as directed and not rely on them as a long-term solution. It is always best to consult with a healthcare provider before starting any new weight management product.

In conclusion, understanding the different types of weight management products available can help you make informed decisions about which may be best for you. Whether you choose supplements, meal replacement shakes, or appetite suppressants, it is important to remember that these products are meant to supplement a healthy diet and exercise routine. By incorporating these products into a comprehensive weight management plan, you can increase your chances of success and achieve your goals in a safe and sustainable way.

Researching and Choosing the Right Products for You

When it comes to weight management, choosing the right products can make a huge difference in your success. Researching and selecting the best products for your individual needs is crucial to achieving your health and fitness goals. With so many options available on the market, it can be overwhelming to know where to start. However, by following a few simple steps, you can make informed decisions that will set you on the path to success.

The first step in researching and choosing the right products for you is to identify your specific weight management goals. Are you looking to lose weight, build muscle, or simply maintain your current weight? Understanding your goals will help you narrow down your options and focus on products that align with your objectives. By setting clear goals, you can make more targeted choices that will support your overall health and well-being.

Once you have established your goals, the next step is to research different weight management products that are available. This may include supplements, meal replacement shakes, exercise equipment, or meal plans. Take the time to read reviews, compare prices, and consult with health professionals to determine which products are best suited to your needs. Remember, what works for one person may not work for another, so it's important to find products that are tailored to your individual preferences and lifestyle.

When selecting weight management products, it's important to consider factors such as ingredients, effectiveness, and safety. Look for products that are made with high-quality, natural ingredients and have been proven to deliver results. Additionally, be wary of products that make unrealistic claims or promises of quick fixes. Remember, sustainable weight management requires a balanced approach that includes healthy eating habits, regular exercise, and consistency.

In conclusion, researching and choosing the right products for your weight management journey is a key component of achieving success. By setting clear goals, conducting thorough research, and considering important factors such as ingredients and safety, you can make informed decisions that will support your overall health and well-being. Remember, it's important to be patient and realistic in your expectations, as sustainable weight management takes time and dedication. With the right products and a positive mindset, you can take on the 30-Day Weight Management Challenge and achieve lasting results.

Incorporating Weight Management Products into Your Routine

Incorporating weight management products into your daily routine can be a game-changer in achieving your health and fitness goals. Whether you're looking to lose weight, gain muscle, or simply maintain a healthy weight, these products can provide the extra support you need to stay on track. By incorporating these products into your routine, you can boost your metabolism, increase energy levels, and improve overall well-being.

One of the most popular weight management products on the market is meal replacement shakes. These convenient shakes are packed with essential nutrients and protein, making them a great option for busy individuals on the go. By replacing one or two meals a day with a shake, you can easily control your calorie intake and ensure you're getting the nutrition your body needs to thrive. Plus, they come in a variety of flavors, so you can find one that suits your taste preferences.

Another effective weight management product to consider is a fat burner supplement. These supplements work by increasing your metabolism and helping your body burn fat more efficiently. When combined with a healthy diet and regular exercise, fat burners can help you reach your weight loss goals faster. Just be sure to choose a reputable brand and follow the recommended dosage for best results.

In addition to meal replacement shakes and fat burners, there are a variety of other weight management products to explore, such as appetite suppressants, metabolism boosters, and meal prep kits. By incorporating a combination of these products into your routine, you can create a personalized plan that works best for your individual needs and goals. Remember, consistency is key when it comes to achieving lasting results, so stick with your routine and stay committed to your health and wellness journey.

Overall, incorporating weight management products into your routine can provide the extra support you need to reach your health and fitness goals. Whether you're looking to lose weight, build muscle, or simply maintain a healthy weight, there are products available to help you along the way. Remember to consult with your healthcare provider before starting any new supplement regimen, and always listen to your body's needs. With dedication, consistency, and the right products, you can achieve the results you desire and live a healthier, happier life.

Chapter 5: Overcoming Challenges and Obstacles

Dealing with Cravings and Emotional Eating

Dealing with cravings and emotional eating can be a challenging aspect of weight management for many men and women aged 20 to 50. It's common to turn to food as a source of comfort or stress relief, but this can often lead to overeating and weight gain. In order to successfully navigate these cravings and emotional triggers, it's important to develop healthy coping mechanisms and strategies.

One effective way to combat cravings and emotional eating is to identify the root cause of these behaviors. Are you eating out of boredom, stress, sadness, or another emotion? Once you understand why you are turning to food, you can begin to address those underlying emotions in a healthier way. This might involve finding alternative activities to distract yourself, such as going for a walk, practicing mindfulness, or talking to a friend.

Another helpful strategy is to practice mindful eating. This involves paying attention to your body's hunger and fullness cues, as well as savoring each bite of food. By slowing down and being present while eating, you are more likely to make conscious choices about what and how much you are consuming. This can help prevent mindless snacking and overeating in response to emotional triggers.

It's also important to have a plan in place for when cravings strike. Stock your kitchen with healthy snacks and meals that you enjoy, so you are less tempted to reach for unhealthy options. Additionally, consider keeping a food journal to track your eating habits and identify patterns that may be contributing to your cravings. By being proactive and prepared, you can better manage your cravings and make healthier choices.

Remember, it's okay to indulge in treats occasionally, but moderation is key. If you find yourself struggling with cravings or emotional eating, don't be too hard on yourself. Weight management is a journey, and setbacks are a normal part of the process. Stay positive, stay focused, and keep working towards your goals. With determination and dedication, you can overcome cravings and emotional eating to achieve lasting weight management success.

Staying Motivated Throughout the 30-Day Challenge

Staying motivated throughout the 30-day weight management challenge can be a challenging task, but with the right mindset and tools, you can achieve your goals. It's important to remember that this journey is not just about losing weight, but about taking control of your health and well-being. By staying motivated, you can set yourself up for long-term success and a healthier lifestyle.

One way to stay motivated throughout the challenge is to set realistic and achievable goals. It's important to break down your overall goal into smaller, more manageable tasks that you can accomplish each day. By setting achievable goals, you can track your progress and celebrate your successes along the way. Remember, small victories lead to big results!

Another key to staying motivated is to surround yourself with a supportive community. Whether it's joining a weight management group, finding an accountability partner, or simply sharing your progress with friends and family, having a support system can make all the difference. By connecting with others who are on a similar journey, you can stay motivated and inspired to keep pushing forward.

It's also important to stay positive and focused on your end goal. Remember why you started this challenge in the first place and visualize the results you want to achieve. By staying positive and focused, you can overcome any obstacles that come your way and stay motivated to reach your goals.

Lastly, don't forget to reward yourself along the way. Celebrate your achievements, no matter how small, and treat yourself to something special as a reward for your hard work. By staying motivated and rewarding yourself for your efforts, you can stay on track and make lasting changes to your health and well-being. Remember, you are capable of achieving anything you set your mind to – stay motivated and keep pushing forward!

Handling Setbacks and Moving Forward

Setbacks are a natural part of any weight management journey, but how we handle them can make all the difference in our success. When faced with a setback, it's important to remember that it's just a temporary obstacle on the path to achieving your goals. Instead of getting discouraged, use setbacks as opportunities to learn and grow. Reflect on what may have led to the setback and think about how you can make positive changes moving forward.

One key to handling setbacks is to stay positive and keep a growth mindset. Instead of beating yourself up over a slip-up, focus on what you can do differently next time. Remember that progress is not always linear, and setbacks are a natural part of the journey. By staying positive and resilient, you'll be better equipped to overcome obstacles and keep moving forward towards your goals.

Another important aspect of handling setbacks is to seek support from others. Whether it's a friend, family member, or support group, having someone to lean on during tough times can make all the difference. Surround yourself with people who will lift you up and encourage you to keep going, even when things get tough. Remember, you're not alone in this journey, and there are people who want to see you succeed.

In addition to seeking support from others, it's important to practice self-compassion and forgiveness. Be kind to yourself and remember that everyone makes mistakes. Instead of dwelling on past setbacks, focus on the present moment and what you can do right now to get back on track. By showing yourself grace and forgiveness, you'll be better able to move forward with confidence and determination.

Remember, setbacks are temporary, but your commitment to your goals is what will ultimately lead to success. Stay positive, seek support, and practice self-compassion as you navigate through challenges. By staying resilient and focused on the bigger picture, you'll be able to overcome setbacks and keep moving forward towards achieving your weight management goals.

Chapter 6: Celebrating Your Success

Reflecting on Your Achievements During the Challenge

Congratulations on completing the 30-Day Weight Management Challenge! Take a moment to reflect on all that you have achieved during this journey. Whether you reached your goal weight, improved your eating habits, or adopted a more active lifestyle, you should be proud of your accomplishments. Remember, progress is progress, no matter how small it may seem.

As you reflect on your achievements, think about the changes you have made and how they have impacted your overall well-being. Have you noticed any improvements in your energy levels, mood, or confidence? Maybe you have received compliments from friends and family on your transformation. Celebrate these victories and use them as motivation to continue on your path to a healthier lifestyle.

It's important to recognize the hard work and dedication that you have put into this challenge. Making changes to your diet and exercise routine can be challenging, but you have shown that you are capable of overcoming obstacles and reaching your goals. Give yourself credit for your commitment and determination, and know that you are capable of achieving anything you set your mind to.

As you look back on the past 30 days, consider what strategies and habits have worked best for you. Maybe you found that meal prepping on Sundays helped you stay on track with your eating goals, or that scheduling workouts in the morning increased your consistency with exercise. Take note of these successful tactics and continue to incorporate them into your daily routine moving forward.

Remember, this is just the beginning of your journey to better health and wellness. Use this reflection period to set new goals for yourself and create a plan for how you will continue to progress on your weight management journey. Stay positive, stay focused, and most importantly, believe in yourself. You have already proven that you have what it takes to succeed – now go out there and make it happen!

Setting New Goals for Continued Weight Management

Congratulations on completing the 30-Day Weight Management Challenge! You have taken the first step towards achieving your health and wellness goals, and now it's time to set new goals for continued weight management. Setting new goals is essential to maintaining your progress and staying motivated on your journey to a healthier lifestyle.

One of the key aspects of setting new goals for continued weight management is to focus on sustainable changes. Instead of aiming for quick fixes or drastic measures, think about small, achievable goals that you can work towards over time. This could include incorporating more fruits and vegetables into your diet, increasing your daily water intake, or adding in regular exercise to your routine.

It's also important to track your progress as you work towards your new goals. Keeping a food journal, logging your workouts, or using a fitness tracker can help you stay accountable and see how far you've come. Celebrate your milestones along the way, whether it's losing a few pounds, fitting into a smaller size, or completing a challenging workout. Remember, progress is progress no matter how small!

Another important aspect of setting new goals for continued weight management is to stay flexible and adjust your goals as needed. Life can be unpredictable, and there may be times when you face setbacks or obstacles. Instead of getting discouraged, use these moments as opportunities to reevaluate your goals and make adjustments that work for you. Remember, it's about progress, not perfection.

In conclusion, setting new goals for continued weight management is an important part of your health and wellness journey. By focusing on sustainable changes, tracking your progress, celebrating your milestones, and staying flexible, you can continue to make positive strides towards a healthier lifestyle. Remember, you have already proven that you have the determination and dedication to succeed – keep up the great work!

Maintaining Your Progress Beyond the 30 Days

Congratulations on completing the 30-Day Weight Management Challenge! You have made significant progress towards your health and fitness goals, and it is important to maintain this momentum beyond the initial 30 days. In this subchapter, we will discuss strategies to help you continue your progress and make lasting lifestyle changes.

One of the key ways to maintain your progress beyond the 30 days is to continue following the healthy habits you have established during the challenge. This includes eating a balanced diet, exercising regularly, and staying hydrated. By making these habits a part of your daily routine, you will be more likely to sustain your weight loss and overall health improvements.

It is also important to set new goals for yourself to stay motivated and continue making progress. Whether it's increasing your daily step count, trying a new fitness class, or setting a target weight to reach, having something to work towards will help keep you on track. Remember, progress is not always linear, and it's okay to have setbacks. The key is to stay focused and resilient in the face of challenges.

In addition to maintaining healthy habits and setting new goals, it is important to seek support from friends, family, or a support group. Having a strong support system can help you stay accountable, provide encouragement, and offer guidance when needed. Surround yourself with positive influences who will help you stay motivated and on track towards your health and fitness goals.

Lastly, remember to celebrate your successes along the way. Acknowledge the progress you have made, no matter how small, and give yourself credit for your hard work. By staying positive and focused on your goals, you will be able to maintain your progress beyond the 30 days and continue on your journey towards a healthier, happier you.

Chapter 7: Conclusion

Final Thoughts and Encouragement for Your Weight Management Journey

Congratulations on completing the 30-day weight management challenge! You have taken the first step towards achieving your health and fitness goals, and I am so proud of you for committing to this journey. Remember, weight management is not just about the number on the scale, but about feeling confident and healthy in your own skin. Keep up the great work and continue to prioritize your well-being.

As you reflect on the past 30 days, remember to celebrate your successes, no matter how small they may seem. Whether you lost a few pounds, made healthier food choices, or incorporated more physical activity into your routine, every positive change is a step in the right direction. Be proud of yourself for making progress and staying dedicated to your goals.

Moving forward, I encourage you to continue practicing the healthy habits you have developed during the challenge. Consistency is key when it comes to weight management, so make sure to stay committed to your nutrition and exercise routines. Remember that progress takes time, and it's okay to have setbacks along the way. The important thing is to stay focused and motivated to keep pushing forward.

It's also essential to listen to your body and prioritize self-care throughout your weight management journey. Make sure to get enough rest, stay hydrated, and manage stress levels to support your overall well-being. Remember that taking care of yourself is not selfish – it is necessary for your physical and mental health. You deserve to feel your best, so don't forget to prioritize self-care as you continue on your path to a healthier lifestyle.

In closing, I want to remind you that you are capable of achieving your weight management goals. Believe in yourself, stay positive, and never give up on your journey to better health. Surround yourself with supportive friends and family members who encourage you to be your best self. You have the strength and determination to succeed, so keep pushing forward and embracing the changes you are making for a healthier, happier you. Good luck on the rest of your weight management journey – I am rooting for you all the way!

Resources for Ongoing Support and Guidance

Congratulations on completing the 30-Day Weight Management Challenge! You have taken a big step towards achieving your health and fitness goals. However, the journey doesn't end here. It is important to have ongoing support and guidance to maintain your progress and continue making positive changes in your life.

There are many resources available to help you stay on track with your weight management goals. One option is to join a support group or community of like-minded individuals who are also working towards improving their health. These groups can provide motivation, accountability, and valuable tips and advice to help you stay focused and motivated.

Another valuable resource for ongoing support and guidance is a health and wellness coach. A coach can work with you one-on-one to create a personalized plan that fits your individual needs and goals. They can provide encouragement, accountability, and guidance to help you overcome any obstacles that may arise on your journey to better health.

Additionally, there are numerous weight management products and tools available to help you stay on track. From fitness trackers and meal planning apps to portion control plates and healthy recipe books, there are many resources to help you make healthy choices and stay motivated. These products can help you stay organized, track your progress, and make healthy living easier and more enjoyable.

Remember, the key to long-term success with weight management is consistency and perseverance. By utilizing the resources available to you for ongoing support and guidance, you can continue making positive changes in your life and achieve your health and fitness goals. Keep up the great work and remember that you are capable of achieving anything you set your mind to!

Taking the Next Steps Towards a Healthier Lifestyle

Congratulations on completing the first 30 days of the weight management challenge! You have taken the first step towards a healthier lifestyle, and now it's time to keep the momentum going. In this chapter, we will discuss the next steps you can take to continue your journey towards better health and wellness.

One of the most important things you can do to maintain a healthy lifestyle is to establish a routine. This means setting aside time each day for exercise, meal planning, and self-care. By creating a schedule and sticking to it, you will be more likely to stay on track with your weight management goals.

Another key aspect of a healthy lifestyle is making smart food choices. This includes eating a balanced diet that is rich in fruits, vegetables, whole grains, and lean proteins. It's also important to limit your intake of processed foods, sugary drinks, and unhealthy fats. By fueling your body with nutritious foods, you will have more energy, feel better overall, and be better equipped to reach your weight management goals.

In addition to eating well, regular exercise is essential for maintaining a healthy weight. Aim to get at least 30 minutes of moderate exercise each day, whether it's going for a walk, hitting the gym, or taking a fitness class. Not only will regular exercise help you burn calories and build muscle, but it will also improve your mood and reduce stress.

Lastly, remember that progress takes time and consistency. It's important to be patient with yourself and celebrate small victories along the way. By staying committed to your health and wellness goals, you will be well on your way to achieving long-term success in managing your weight and living a healthier lifestyle. Keep up the great work!